Frankincense Oil

Everything You Need To Know About The
Essential Oil Fit For Kings

By Amy Joyson

Disclaimer – Please read!

The information provided in this book is designed to provide helpful information on the subjects discussed. This book is not meant to be used, nor should it be used, to diagnose or treat any medical condition. For diagnosis or treatment of any medical problem, consult your own physician. The publisher and author are not responsible for any specific health or allergy needs that may require medical supervision and are not liable for any damages or negative consequences from any treatment, action, application or preparation, to any person reading or following the information in this book. References are provided for informational purposes only and do not constitute endorsement of any websites or other sources. Readers should be aware that the websites listed in this book may change.

Table of Contents

Frankincense Oil Blend Remedies/Recipes...............42

Introduction

Thank you for joining me for another instalment in this comprehensive series on various essential oils and their wondrous therapeutic potentials! The focus of this book will be frankincense, one of the most prized and revered essential oils across the ages. It holds such an important place in both the modern world of aromatherapy, as well as in pre-modern medicine and religion, that it has often been referred to as the 'king of kings' of essential oils. The following guide will take a look at the story of frankincense – this 'king of kings' – and provide the reader with everything they need to know about its remarkable healing properties and therapeutic powers.

For those accustomed with the layout of previous books in this series, this guide will follow a similar format as our earlier instalments. We will begin with an exploration of the storied and colorful history of frankincense, including a look at perhaps the most famous written reference to the prized commodity. This will be followed by an examination of the key properties and chemical composition of frankincense – that is, how and why this therapeutic agent acts in the remarkable way that it does. Next, we will take a look at tips on extracting frankincense oil at home, including best practice and recommended safety precautions. Also discussed are general safety precautions to be observed when using essential oils, as well as some general advice on how essential oils may be administered.

In the latter half of this book, we will round out our guide on frankincense with a breakdown of detailed information on the therapeutic potential of the oil, starting with a summary of the key health benefits of frankincense and continuing with a comprehensive collection of remedies and recipes that make use of frankincense – either as the sole or primary ingredient.

In its entirety, the principal aim for this book is that it might act as a kind of 'masterclass' for those wishing to educate themselves on the topic of frankincense oil. From everything you need to know about the background, key properties, extraction and application of this therapeutic agent, this guide is useful both as a 'complete' education on frankincense, as well as a quick reference for all things related to this wonderful essential oil. This guide will cover some of the similar themes and content from previous books, but with a specific reference to frankincense. If you're a newcomer to this series, don't worry – the content is constructed in such a way that it is suitable for both complete novices and aromatherapy experts alike!

With this in mind, we hope you enjoy everything that the following guide has to offer, and that you take from it everything you need to know about the marvelous frankincense. So sit back, relax (and perhaps burn some wonderfully fragrant frankincense incense while you read!) as we take a journey through the remarkable and mystical world of frankincense.

Origin/History of Frankincense Essential Oil

"And going into the house they saw the child with Mary his mother, and they fell down and worshiped him. Then, opening their treasures, they offered him gifts, gold and frankincense and myrrh." (Matthew 2:11)

Frankincense oil is derived from the aromatic resin of four different species of tree or shrub in the Boswellia family. These include the *Boswellia sacra, Boswellia frereana, Boswellia serrata* and *Boswellia papyrifera,* with the first being the most common source of frankincense and is typically the variety from which therapeutic quality frankincense is obtained. Most species are geographically limited to the area of Southern Arabia and Northeast Africa thanks to the unique seasonal climate typical of the area (although some species can also be found on the Indian subcontinent and southern China, discussed further below). The traditional name for frankincense is *'olibanum'*, which is understood to be derived from the Arabic *'al-lubbān'*, meaning 'that which results from milking'. This seemingly obscure eponym actually refers to the method by which frankincense is obtained, via the 'milking' of the Boswellia tree. This extraction technique involves making relatively shallow horizontal cuttings in the bark of the tree, which expose a porous layer in the wood a few centimeters beneath the surface. This allows for the milky resin of the plant to slowly seep through the veins of the tree to this newly exposed surface, crystallizing in teardrop formations over the course of about a week. The 'cutting' process is repeated another two or three times until the finest quality frankincense, found deep within the tree, eventually seeps to the surface. After some time the crystallized resin is then harvested and further dried and hardened (typically in a cool, dark place such as the sheltered ledge of a cave) to produce the final product – a commodity so precious that it is sometimes referred to as the 'pearls of the desert'. The oil of frankincense may then be obtained via the steam distillation of this hardened resin. Frankincense resin and its oil have been produced in the manner for thousands of years, from ancient times through to the present day.

There are few essential oils that are able to boast the same rich and storied history as that of frankincense. Frankincense was long highly valued throughout much of the ancient world, a fact which is evidenced by the sheer volume of citations which refer to the prized commodity. Perhaps the most famous of these can be found in the New Testament account of the birth of the baby Jesus, found in Matthew and quoted above, wherein frankincense was storied to be one among three of some of the most expensive luxury items of the age that were gifted by the 'Magi' to the new born Messiah. However, there are many, many more accounts of this widely revered aromatic compound that can be found in a range of historical sources. There are many more references to frankincense throughout the Bible, namely in the Talmud book of Leviticus, which hint at the sacred properties assigned to the commodity by those of the Jewish faith. Famed Roman author and naturalist Pliny the Elder noted preciousness of frankincense, identified the agent as an antidote to hemlock poisoning (which, as an aside, had been the method by which Greek philosopher Socrates committed suicide), and claimed that the valued export had made Southern Arabia – from whence frankincense was sourced – the richest land on Earth.

Frankincense has been harvested and exported by the peoples of Southern Arabia and exported to various cultures throughout Europe, Asia and Africa for several thousands of years. Records indicate that frankincense was first produced there as far back as 7,000 B.C.E. The Babylonians and Assyrians are believed to have used frankincense during religious ceremonies, while in Ancient Egypt, the commodity was bought by the shipload for a variety of practical and spiritual applications. There, frankincense was used as part of the preparation for the ritual purification and embalming of mummified pharaohs, as well as in the worship of the gods Ra and Horus, and was also used for cosmetic purposes. Evidence of the revered place of frankincense in Egyptian life and ritual can be found in illustrations found on the walls of the temple of Queen Hatshepsut (who died in 1458 B.C.E.), which depict sacks of prized frankincense resin being imported from the Land of Punt. Meanwhile, the Greeks and the Romans also imported massive quantities of the resin, which was burned as incense during religious ceremonies and festivals, as well as during the process of cremation, and was also applied for a number of different therapeutic remedies. The infamous Roman Emperor Nero is said to have ordered an entire year's harvest of frankincense to be burned at the funeral of a favored mistress, a display typical of his reputed tendency towards excess.

Given the extremely high value attributed to frankincense products throughout the ancient world, various efforts were made to challenge the monopoly that kingdoms of Southern Arabia have had in controlling the frankincense market. So prized was the commodity in the Roman Empire, that Augustus Caesar dispatched around 10,000 troops in an ultimately failed attempt to seize control of the frankincense market at the source. Historically, more lateral attempts have been made to wrest control of the Arabian frankincense cartel with efforts to grow species from the *Boswellia* genus in other parts of the world, including the Levant in the Middle East. Ultimately, the bulk of these attempts have typically ended in failure. One notable exception to this experience, however, can be found in Southern China, where frankincense has been grown and used extensively in traditional medicine for centuries. There, the extract of frankincense oil has been used to remedy a range of therapeutic complaints; from encouraging the flow of spiritual energy, to the relief of general pain, and even the treatment of cancer. Also in the East, frankincense has a long history of medicinal use in Ayurvedic Indian culture.

In the transition from the classical era to the dark ages, the trade in frankincense petered out dramatically in the West. The main obstacle to the trade in frankincense came with the prohibition of the use of incense during services by the early Catholic Church. Although the Church later lifted this restriction, the original edict saw frankincense all but disappear from the European continent for a brief period. After being effectively lost to Western civilization for many years, the Middle Ages saw Frankish Crusaders reintroduce frankincense as an important commodity in the European continent. Contrary to popular belief, however, the etymology of the product's English name is not owed to these religious warriors. Instead, the name comes from the Old French, *'franc encens'*, which roughly translates to 'incense of a very high quality'. In any event, frankincense soon saw a return to glory in the west as a highly prized commodity and was sought after during this time for use in religious rites and ceremonies, as an agent for perfumery, and in medicine.

In more recent times, frankincense has received a lot of attention from the scientific community, which has sought to verify the ancient claims that frankincense is a panacea for many ills. And interestingly, much of this research has indeed supported the seemingly folkloric reputation of frankincense as a remedial miracle. Various studies (which will be highlighted later in this book) have highlighted the mechanisms by which frankincense has a therapeutic effect on the human body – from its anti-inflammatory and analgesic qualities, through to its ability to act as a natural anti-depressant. Such is the interest and potential in the healing power of frankincense, that research has even ventured into the world of oncology and everlasting efforts to find an elusive cure for cancer.

So it would seem that frankincense has long captivated great civilizations, from the era of the ancients, through to the modern age of science. Interestingly, while it was accepted by cultures thousands of years into the past that frankincense contains remarkable therapeutic qualities, we are only now just learning to reconcile the healing power of frankincense with the empiricism of modern medicine. As part of a revolution in science and medicine, we are beginning to re-learn that the incredible design of nature holds the key to solving many of our most feared pathologies and complex medical puzzles.

The Key Properties Of Frankincense Essential Oil

The chemical composition of frankincense oil

With an understanding of the historical context and application of frankincense in mind we will turn briefly to an examination of the chemical makeup of the oil. Frankincense oil boasts a number of unique remedial properties that can be used to greatly improve or enhance one's well-being. These special qualities are made possible by the distinct chemical profile of frankincense oil, which we will now explore in some detail.

The resin of the *Boswellia sacra* (the main species from which frankincense oil is derived) is understood to contain dozens of unique chemical constituents. In order of percentage by volume, the main compounds found in frankincense oil include: α-pinene (~68%), limonene+β-phellandrene (~6%), sabinene (~3%), β-pinene (~2%), camphene (~2%), myrcene (~1%) and α-thujene (<1%). However, there is a significant amount of variation in terms of the specific composition of a given sample of frankincense oil. The main factors which influence this variation are the quality of the oil that is sampled, but perhaps more significantly, the species of Boswellia from which the frankincense has been obtained. To cite an empirical example of this variation in chemical composition, we can compare the main compounds found in the frankincense producing species *Boswellia carterii,* which has the following composition (again in order of percentage by volume): α-pinene (~37%), limonene+β-phellandrene (~14%), α-thujene (~8%), myrcene (~7%), sabinene (~5%), β-pinene (~2%) and camphene (~1%).

Upon closer examination, we can see that the main compounds found in frankincense oils are a class of aromatic compounds known as monoterpenes. As shown above, the monoterpene α-pinene is the primary constituent in most variants of frankincense oil, while others, including limonene, β-pinene and sabinene, all play a prominent role in lending the essence many of its unique therapeutic properties. These extremely complex organic compounds also give frankincense its distinctive fruity, woody aroma. Also found in smaller, but still significant concentrations in frankincense oil are boswellic acids, which have been shown in clinical research to exhibit notable and distinct therapeutic properties, including anti-inflammatory, analgesic and anti-rheumatic effects. Some of these will be discussed further later in this chapter.

The A to Z of frankincense oil's therapeutic properties

It is no surprise that frankincense has been held in such high regard for its therapeutic properties for more than 5,000 years. What's more, not only are the accounts of the healing power of frankincense anecdotal; rather, many of the purported therapeutic benefits of the aromatic resin have been reinforced by clinical research. The following section will highlight these remarkable attributes and attempt to highlight the true usefulness of the essence of frankincense as a panacea for a range of ills.

Antiseptic: As with many essential oils, frankincense exhibits a powerful antiseptic quality, which makes it a great agent for the treatment of superficial cuts or wounds. This property sees frankincense oil create an inhospitable environment for bacteria and other pathogens, killing germs that come into direct contact with the essence. In particular, the potent antibacterial and antiviral properties of the essence (discussed below) make frankincense a particularly effective antiseptic agent.

Analgesic: Frankincense has been shown in clinical conditions to be an effective agent for pain relief. Clinical research indicates that this analgesic property is largely thought to be thanks to the presence of a range of boswellic acids which exhibit potent analgesic effect. An analysis of frankincense oil derived from *Boswellia serrata* indicates that one of the most significant such acids found in this species is 3-O-acetyl-11-keto-beta-boswellic acid – more simply abbreviated as 'AKBA'. This 'AKBA' compound has been isolated in a clinical environment and has, in some cases, been found to be as effective in treating pain and inflammation as traditional drugs such as ibuprofen. It is understood to work by blocking enzymes that are involved in driving the body's natural inflammation response.

Anti-depressant: Frankincense oil has also been shown to have some effectiveness in alleviating depression. A joint research study conducted between Johns Hopkins University and the Hebrew University in Jerusalem showed that burning incense was found to have a positive effect in alleviating mood and easing depression. The study saw a compound found in frankincense, *incensole acetate*, isolated and administered to mice. It was found that areas of the brain and nerve circuits in the mice that typically responded to traditional anti-depressants and other psychoactive drugs (including benzodiazepines, which are typically prescribed to combat anxiety) were similarly affected by the frankincense derivative.

Anti-fungal: Certain species of *Boswellia* (including *Boswellia carterii)* have been shown in clinical settings to have a significant anti-fungal effect. This makes frankincense oils useful for a range of anti-fungal treatments, from candida to ringworm.

Anti-inflammatory: Frankincense is one of a number of essential oils that has been shown to have good effect in inhibiting the body's inflammation response. This, in part, makes it a good agent for the treatment of superficial wounds, as well as for inflammatory disorders in different parts of the body. As discussed above, the main agent believed to be responsible for this anti-inflammatory effect is the boswellic acid 'AKBA', which has been shown to be, in some cases, as effective as traditional anti-inflammatory drugs such as ibuprofen.

Anti-rheumatic: Further to the anti-inflammatory property of frankincense, the essential oil of frankincense is effective in the treatment of rheumatological disorders, such as gout or arthritis. Again, clinical research has demonstrated the efficacy of frankincense as a therapeutic agent in this particular area. An Indian study determined that, in a sample of 50 osteoarthritic patients suffering knee-joint inflammation, those who were administered a remedy containing frankincense enjoyed significant improvements in terms of pain, inflammation and function. Specifically, they reported up to 70 percent better knee-joint mobility and a greater than 50 percent reduction in swelling. This effect is believed to be due to the presence of the abovementioned AKBA molecule, as well as other anti-inflammatory boswellic acids.

Antiviral: With the ability to kill a number of different pathogenic viral strains, frankincense exhibits powerful antiviral properties. This quality again makes it a suitable agent for treating cuts and wounds, as well as for combating other viral based conditions, such as influenza, warts and herpes. Again, clinical research has been carried out which supports the hypothesis that frankincense exhibits antiviral properties.

Bactericide: In addition to being a powerful antiviral agent, frankincense is also exhibits potent anti-bacterial properties.

This makes it a suitable agent for keeping superficial wounds from succumbing to bacterial infection, and can also be effective in treating respiratory infections (for example). Clinical research has shown that certain species of *Boswellia* (notably, *Boswellia sacra*) significantly inhibit bacterial growth in a controlled laboratory environment.

Carminative: As a carminative agent, frankincense works to reduce to production of gas within the digestive tract. Treatment with frankincense can therefore help to eliminate gas, reduce abdominal bloating, and alleviate indigestion and flatulence.

Cicatrisant: As a cicatrisant, frankincense encourages the generation of scar tissue which aids greatly with the healing of wounds.

Cytophylactic: With the ability to encourage the growth of new skin cells, frankincense can help to repair wounds, heal scars and other skin damage, and reduce the appearance of ageing.

Deodorant: The pleasant, woody/fruity aroma of frankincense oil, combined with its antimicrobial properties makes for a good active ingredient in a natural deodorant. These properties mean that frankincense can either be used alone or in conjunction with other complementary aromatic oils for this purpose.

Digestive: Frankincense facilitates digestion by encouraging the secretion of digestive juices and controls inflammation in the digestive system. This makes it a useful treatment when suffering from the discomfort associated with poor digestion, and a good alternative to commercially available antacids.

Diuretic: For those wishing to either detoxify the body of impurities or purge excess water weight, frankincense is a suitable agent thanks to its properties as a diuretic.

Emmenagogue: Frankincense can be a boon when it comes to stimulating menstruation, which can be useful in the event of amenorrhea (absence of regular menstrual flow). This property also serves to alleviate many of the adverse symptoms associated with menstruation, such as cramping. Please note, the emmenagogue properties of frankincense also mean that its use should be avoided by pregnant women as it may stimulate early labor.

Expectorant: As an expectorant, frankincense can aid in the expulsion of mucous from the airways. This is useful in helping to clear respiratory infections and colds and viruses that have spread to the chest.

Sedative: Frankincense can act as a powerful sedative, which has a number of practical applications. It can be used to relax and calm the mind; alleviate stress and anxiety; and even help to regulate breathing and normalize elevated blood pressure.

Uterine: As a uterine, frankincense is a useful agent for maintaining good uterine health. It can encourage healthy blood flow to the area, regulate hormonal balance, and prevent the development of uterine cysts. Anecdotal accounts suggest that frankincense may be used successfully to alleviate some of the symptoms associated with endometriosis.

Vulnerary: Frankincense can help to speed the healing of both internal and external wounds, thanks to its remarkable powers as a vulnerary agent. Its proven ability to inhibit the growth of bacterial and viral infections, along with its wound repairing qualities make frankincense a notable entry in this category.

Frankincense Oil Extraction

As stated in earlier chapters, frankincense is sourced from several species of tree/shrub within the *Boswellia* family. All are native to Southern Arabia, India, Northeast Africa and the Red Sea region, and depend on the unique climactic conditions of the area for their successful growth and optimal yield of resin. Very hot desert conditions, contrasted by the extreme rainfall associated with the monsoon season, are the specific parameters which see this region enjoy its position as the home of frankincense. Because of these unique conditions, it is unusual to find frankincense sourced from other geographical areas. And for this reason, one is unlikely to be able to grow *Boswellia* trees and source their frankincense resin locally (unless your home can be found in Yemen, Oman, or perhaps, Somalia!). However, it is nonetheless possible to obtain your frankincense oil by extraction from frankincense resin crystals, which the following chapter will explore in some detail.

Frankincense can be obtained in a range of qualities: from the very purest, clear/silvery resin, to a lower grade product that is typically cloudier and darker in colour, and is broken into very small, hard pieces. As a rule, the highest quality frankincense resin is typically that sourced from Oman or Yemen; perhaps the biggest single customer for frankincense today is the Catholic Church, which typically uses the cheaper and lower quality Somalian product. As is the logical rule with all essential oil extractions, a higher quality of raw material will yield a higher quality essence. For this reason, cheaper frankincense oil – though it may be found – is often derived from a resin of inferior quality.

While it is possible to purchase superior quality frankincense oil from certain reputable vendors, it can be difficult to assess the quality of frankincense essence once it has been extracted from frankincense crystals. There are few tell-tale visual indicators that can be relied upon for proof of the quality of most essential oils; instead, advanced and expensive chemical analysis is necessary to make such an assessment of a refined essence. As such, one of the few ways to be certain of the quality of frankincense oil is to visually assess the quality of frankincense resin from which the eponymous oil is to be derived, and carry out the extraction from this raw material locally and independently. Fortunately, as frankincense oil is typically extracted through the method of steam distillation, it can be relatively easily done at home given the availability of the right equipment.

Steam distillation basics

Steam distillation involves, as the name suggests, the use of steam to draw out the volatile compounds contained within organic matter, and cooling and condensing the resulting steam vapor. This method is fairly common when it comes to extracting essential oils, and is indeed the process by which frankincense oil is best obtained. The chief requirement in this process is a home still, which can be easily assembled in an *ad-hoc* fashion using individual components or, even more simply, with the purchase of a complete pre-fabricated still. Those with a little technical nous may wish to construct a still of their own making; this section is for these ambitious folk and others who simply wish to know more about the extraction process!

The simplest type of homemade still is what is known as a pot still. This type of system is perfect for the extraction of frankincense oil from frankincense resin. It consists of three main components: the *pot*, or boiler, in which the raw material and steam source is contained; the *condenser*, which cools the steam to return it to a liquid state; and the *essencier*, in which the essential oil is collected and separated from other compounds. First of all, the pot should be quite large; big enough to comfortably hold a substantial amount of raw material (somewhere between one and four kilograms of frankincense resin), as well having as enough space for boiling water at the bottom. The pot should also be tiered to allow for the separation of the raw material from the steam source, and should permit the easy addition of water so that the pot is not at risk of boiling dry during the distillation process. A final important point about the pot is that it should have a tightly sealed lid, so that all steam that comes from the pot will flow directly up through the condenser. Your still *will not* function properly without a tightly fitting lid! Next, the condenser is normally a double-walled length of tubing, which is typically water cooled to permit the condensation process to occur. This typically attaches to the lid of the pot at a tightly sealed outlet, with the other end ending running into the *essencier*. This final piece, the *essencier,* is generally made of glass and is a long vertical tube shape with a tap at the base. All parts are generally best made from heat resistant glass or non-reactive metal, such as stainless steel. Copper is also suitable, however its oxidation may compromise the purity of the final product.

The distillation process

Once the distillation process is underway, it becomes a relatively low maintenance affair which can last for a couple of hours. However, key to a perfect distillation are thorough preparation and close attention. The process begins with the preparation of the raw material. In this case, frankincense resin should be added to the top tier of the pot in a layer no thicker than three inches. This allows for the steam to thoroughly permeate the layer of resin and allows for the optimum yield of oil. (In terms of sourcing frankincense resin for the purpose of distillation, there are a number of vendors who sell this product online; however, it is important to do your research before committing to a purchase and make efforts to buy from reputable sellers.) As mentioned above, the whole distillation process can take a couple of hours, during which time a close eye should be kept on the still. It is important to make sure that the bottom of the pot doesn't boil dry and begin to burn, as this can compromise the whole product – both the resin and the oil – which can be a very costly mistake. It is also important to make sure that the condenser is functioning properly, with cold water running through the outer chamber constantly. If not, this can affect the yield of the final product. As a rule of thumb, the expected yield of frankincense oil from a sample of resin can be anywhere between 2 and 10 percent; generally, a higher quality raw material leans towards the higher end of this spectrum.

As the pot begins to heat, steam will begin to flow up through the condenser, eventually liquefying in the essencier. Therein, one can observe the liquid separating into two distinct layers, with the bulk of the mixture consisting of what is called hydrosol settling at the bottom of the essencier tube, and the less dense frankincense oil floating at the top. (Hydrosol, a byproduct of essential oil extraction, has a range of cosmetic, domestic and therapeutic applications, a number of which can be found discussed in other written resources on aromatherapy, or online.) As mentioned earlier, the entire distillation process can take one to two hours. One can note when the distillation is approaching its final stages, as the yield of liquid dripping into the essencier from the condenser tube begins to slow to a standstill. At this point, the heat source at the pot should be discontinued and the still left to rest for about half an hour, allowing any remaining vapors circulating in the still to be converted into hydrosol/essential oil.

Now, the hydrosol/essential oil can be collected from the essencier. This is done by placing a suitably sized, open-topped receptacle beneath the spout of the essencier and *very slowly* opening the tap. This should be done very cautiously so as to allow *only the hydrosol* to flow into the receptacle. During this process, a close eye should be kept on the level in the essencier where the hydrosol separates from the frankincense oil. As the last of the hydrosol begins to leave the essencier, the tap should almost be completely closed, only allowing a drip at a time to leave the spout. The tap should be shut off completely before any essential oil leaves the essenicer; this is very important, as any oil that runs into the hydrosol at this point will be lost. Finally, with the last step of the process, the tap of the essencier may be re-opened and the frankincense oil collected into a suitably sized vial. Essential oils are best kept in tightly sealed, dark glass vials (or at least, stored in transparent glass in a dark place), which limits the chance of a photochemical reaction occurring while the oil is in storage.

Safety

Steam distillation of essential oils as outlined above is a relatively simple and straightforward process. However, it is vital to operate a still with caution, given the high temperatures involved. As with the use of any process involving a heat source, close attention should be paid to the still during operation to avoid the risk of fire or injury to a third party. Additionally, given that the extraction process involves the generation of steam, one should work with care to avoid direct steam burns. Finally, one should ensure that all equipment used in the distillation process is in good working order, checking that seals are in place and all items are free from defects which may lead to the failure of the still.

Complete Safety With Frankincense Essential Oil

As with the use of practically any essential oil, there are a few key safety precautions to keep in mind when using frankincense oil for therapeutic purposes. Although essential oils are natural and generally safe to use (especially when compared to the artificial chemicals and medicines we often thoughtlessly introduce to our bodies), there are a few situations where they may cause an adverse reaction in a patient. The following chapter will take a look at how to avoid such situations, specifically with regards to frankincense oil.

When it comes to the use of any essential oil in the practice of aromatherapy, one should exercise the same level of caution for each. Fortunately, when it comes to frankincense, it is considered particularly mild when compared to some of the more volatile essential oils available for therapeutic treatment. It may be used safely in most patients and generally has a limited association with inducing adverse reactions. Generally, one should avoid taking essential oils internally as they can lead to irritation or burning of the digestive tract. However, as frankincense oil is listed as an FDA approved food additive and flavoring agent, it may be administered in a diluted oral solution in some cases. Please note, however, that before commencing an orally ingested treatment that contains frankincense oil, you should consult a qualified aromatherapist for advice.

Frankincense oil can be administered in a number of different ways, and most of the treatments outlined in this book can be safely used with most patients. However, there are a few precautions to keep in mind when following the treatments prescribed in this guide. First, it is important to only apply frankincense oil for therapeutic purposes in diluted concentrations. This is because frankincense oil (like all essential oils) contains highly concentrated volatile chemicals, which can cause an adverse skin reaction (including minor burns) in some patients. Although frankincense is considered one of the more mild essential oils and may be applied 'neat' in some cases, this should only be done under the advice or supervision of a qualified aromatherapist. Additionally, before commencing a treatment in which frankincense is to be applied to the skin, it is advisable to test a small patch of skin for sensitivity to the oil before beginning a full treatment. To do so, apply the particular treatment to a small patch of skin on the back of the hand and wait for half an hour to see if any adverse reaction occurs. If no reaction occurs during this time, it is generally consider safe to proceed with a full treatment.

Secondly, when applying any essential oil through massage, it is important to take the medical history and condition of the patient into consideration. Vigorous massage should be avoided in both the very old and very young, as well as in cases where the patient is particularly frail. Additionally, the application of massage should generally be precluded in cases where the patient has tumors, hernias or flesh wounds, and also in cases where a patient has a communicable skin disease (particularly for the safety of the masseur). Of course, a case by case judgment is a good path to take in this regard, and situations where the stimulation of intense massage appears to have the potential to cause harm should be avoided.

Third, due to its classification as an emmenagogue and abortifacient, frankincense should also be avoided for use in pregnant women. This classification means that, while it may be applied in some cases to stimulate uterine function and localized blood flow, frankincense may cause early labor and stimulate abortion. Frankincense may be used in a few cases during pregnancy (e.g. to help induce labor towards the end of a pregnancy), but as a general rule, should be only administered under the direction or supervision of a qualified aromatherapist or physician. If you are uncertain whether a remedy including frankincense is suitable for you, please consult your physician before commencing treatment.

Fourth, further to the ability of frankincense to increase uterine blood flow, it also appears to have a notable effect in boosting circulation by thinning the blood. As a result, frankincense is contraindicated in patients who are either suffering from blood disorders (such as hemophilia), or those already taking drugs which may thin the blood (such as warfarin, ibuprofen or aspirin, for example). Again, if unsure, please consult your doctor before beginning treatment with frankincense.

As a final note on safety while using frankincense oil, it is also important to take into consideration the suitability of other ingredients when using a blend containing frankincense oil. Third party proprietary blends may list frankincense as a main ingredient, but can also contain concentrations of volatile oils or other ingredients that may pose certain health risks in certain patients. For this reason, it is important to be aware of the exact ingredient being used when carrying out an aromatherapy treatment using such a product, and to remain vigilant when it comes to their potential risk.

General Guide to Applying Essential Oils

As with applying all essential oils for therapeutic purposes, there are a few general guidelines that should be observed when administering frankincense oil for therapeutic purposes. Frankincense is generally considered a relatively 'safe' therapeutic agent; it can generally be used in most situations and applications by users with little training in the administration of essential oils. The following chapter will take a look at some of the methods by which frankincense oil may be administered as a therapeutic agent, highlighting some of the advantages and precautions associated with each method.

Topical application

When it comes to aromatherapy, topical application is one of the simplest and most direct methods of receiving therapeutic benefit from an essential oil. When it comes to frankincense, this is perhaps the most useful and common method of administration. Frankincense may be used as an antiseptic ointment, as a topical anti-inflammatory, anti-rheumatic and anti-ageing treatment, and is best administered topically for these types of treatment. As mentioned in the earlier chapter on safety precautions, while frankincense is a relatively mild essential oil and thus, may be applied 'neat' in some circumstances, this should only be done under the guidance of a trained aromatherapist. As a rule, however, topical application of essential oils should only be administered diluted due to the highly concentrated nature of the volatile compounds found within. Topical treatment with frankincense oil can be carried out via basic self-application, massage, or simply added to a bath.

Massage

One of the more popular ways to topically administer essential oils is via massage, and frankincense is no exception to this rule. Some of the advantages offered by massage over other treatments include: the stimulation of blood flow, which speeds the circulation of essential oils through the blood stream; treatment of muscle soreness and localized tension/pain; induced feelings of relaxation; and lowered blood pressure, just to name a few. There are a range of different massage techniques and therapies which can offer different benefits depending on the desired treatment outcome. For example, traditional 'Swedish' massage is useful for general application, treating muscle soreness and encouraging healthy circulation. Meanwhile, a more specialized aromatherapy based treatment, such as the relaxing 'raindrop technique' massage style, is useful for treating stress and inducing relaxation. As highlighted in the earlier chapter on safety precautions, strenuous massage should be avoided in the very old or very young, as well as in frail patients. Additionally, massage is best avoided in those who have tumors local to the massage area, those with a high fever (massage can exacerbate fever related illnesses), and those with communicable skin diseases.

To learn more about the use of massage in aromatherapy treatments, you should consult the earlier guide in this series dedicated to the theme of massage and aromatherapy, which gives detailed advice on different massage techniques, as well as the different treatments and conditions for which aromatherapy massage is a suitable option.

Inhalation

Another great way to administer frankincense therapeutically is via inhalation. Inhalation of fragrant essential oils such as frankincense is perhaps the best way to treat conditions related to mood, emotions and the brain. This is because the olfactory system (which is basically the body's scent processing system) shares close links with the limbic system, or the emotion center of the brain.

In terms of safety precautions, inhalation is perhaps one of the least invasive and safest methods of delivery of an essential oil, as there is little danger of adverse allergic reaction via this method. However, care should be taken when applying direct inhalation of any essential oil, including frankincense, particularly when the patient is suffering from asthma or another intensive respiratory ailment, such as bronchitis. This is because the vapors of the oil may irritate the lungs and cause the airways to close in some severe reactions. In these cases, inhalation treatment is still possible but is best limited to an indirect treatment by using a room diffuser, for example.

Ingestion

Treatment via ingestion of frankincense oil is possible; however, as with therapeutic treatment involving *any* essential oil, this is generally not recommended. This is because the volatile compounds found in all essential oils are highly concentrated and may irritate the sensitive digestive tracts and mucous membranes of some patients. In cases where the oral administration of frankincense oil is recommended, there are some conditions that should be followed. First, frankincense oil should only be taken orally if diluted in water. Generally, the ratio for dilution should be never greater than 10 drops of frankincense oil per liter of water. Second, there are few essential oils that may be taken orally; as such, one should be careful to avoid mixing these with frankincense, in the case that frankincense oil is to be taken orally in a blended solution.

Finally, frankincense oil should only ever be taken orally under the strict advice and supervision of a trained aromatherapist. DO NOT self-prescribe the ingestion of any essential oil without clearance from a trained aromatherapist.

The Health Benefits of Frankincense Oil

Frankincense oil is remarkable in that it has been used for its healing powers by a number of different cultures across several millennia. The following chapter will explore some of the core health benefits associated with frankincense oil, and attempt to unlock the mystery behind some of these key therapeutic attributes.

Pain relief and anti-inflammatory

A study conducted by Professor Dr. Oliver Werz of the Friedrich Schiller University Jena, Germany concluded that "the resin from the trunk of Boswellia trees contains anti-inflammatory substances". Professor Wertz's research isolated and identified boswellic acid as the primary therapeutic component in frankincense oil. Wertz and his research team found that these active ingredients inhibited the body's inflammatory response by interfering with certain mechanisms and pain pathways. Specifically, they found that "[b]oswellic acids interact with several different proteins that are part of inflammatory reactions, but most of all with an enzyme which is responsible for the synthesis of prostaglandin E2, [these] acids block this enzyme efficiently and thereby reduce the inflammatory reaction".

Immunity booster

Another impressive feature of frankincense oil is its apparent ability to fortify the body's natural immune response. Although there is some uncertainty when it comes to pinpointing the chemical agent responsible for this vital effect, it is again believed to be a result of the presence of the impressive boswellic acids, including 'AKBA' and 11-keto-beta-boswellic acid, or 'KBA'. This property has a wide range of potential applications, including fortifying the immunity of those suffering with immune disorders, or simply boosting the immunity of healthy patients to help ward off the common cold.

Antiseptic and disinfectant

As with many other essential oils, frankincense is a very powerful antiseptic agent and disinfectant. This makes it useful in the fight against infection, whether in the form of cleaning wounds, or targeting microbes within the body. Alternatively, this quality also makes frankincense oil a good purificant which can be applied to objects to kill harmful viruses and bacteria.

Cancer fighting agent?

Much has been made in recent years of the potential for frankincense to play a significant role in the treatment of some cancers. Although the clinical evidence needed to thoroughly substantiate these claims is yet to be extended beyond a controlled clinical setting, there are a number of *in vitro* studies which highlight the potential of frankincense as an important link in the ubiquitous fight against cancer. For example, research conducted by the University of Leicester found the abovementioned 'AKBA' compound (present in many variants of frankincense) could be used to successfully target and kill ovarian cancer cells in late-stage ovarian cancer patients. Numerous other studies have been conducted which highlight the potential for 'AKBA' and other volatile constituents found in frankincense oil to destroy different types of cancer cells.

Brain health

There have been several connections made between the use of frankincense and its effect on our mental wellbeing. From ancient times, frankincense has been afforded a sacred quality and closely associated with religious ceremonies and rituals. Recent clinical studies have shown that there may be a good deal of science which supports the idea that frankincense has the power to lift us to a more spiritual plane. As mentioned elsewhere in this guide, one of the leading compounds thought to be responsible for the generally positive effect of frankincense in terms of mental wellbeing is *incensole acetate*. It is suggested that this chemical can have a range of practical influences, including alleviating stress, reducing anxiety and easing depression.

Pure Frankincense Oil Remedies

In the previous chapter we discussed a few of the key areas in which frankincense can have notable therapeutic benefits for the user. This chapter will now explore some of the specific ways in which the essence of frankincense may be applied as the sole active ingredient in a remedy. From stress relief to wound treatment, the following will no doubt prove eye-opening for many amateur aromatherapists in revealing the versatile capabilities of frankincense oil.

Oral hygiene

Frankincense has been used for millennia by various cultures as a means of maintain good oral hygiene. Traditionally, tooth aches, cavities and gum disease have been avoided by chewing the resin of frankincense, releasing the active volatile oils within that kill bacteria and help to fight inflammation. To make your own frankincense based mouthwash, add five drops of frankincense oil to one glass of water and stir well. Rinse mouth with one mouthful of the mouthwash at a time, spitting it into the sink before taking another mouthful. Continue until all of the solution has been used. For best results, perform treatment twice daily.

Antiseptic wound treatment

Further to the potential for frankincense oil to be used for maintaining oral health, it can also be used with great success as a general antiseptic agent. The antimicrobial and antibacterial qualities of the oil help to clean bites, cuts, scrapes and other wounds, and keep them from becoming infected. Meanwhile, the anti-inflammatory and analgesic properties of frankincense help to reduce swelling and ease pain. To treat a wound with frankincense oil, add six drops of the essence of frankincense to 10mL of aloe vera gel and mix thoroughly. The resulting mixture can be applied liberally to wounds as required.

Scar treatment

Interestingly, frankincense can continue to be useful long after a wound has healed. The cytophylactic properties of frankincense help to encourage the growth of new, healthy skin cells, and reduce the appearance of scarring. This treatment can be useful, for example, in reducing the visibility of scars from cuts or stretch marks. To make a frankincense based treatment for scars, combine 10 drops of frankincense oil with 20 mL of coconut oil, and the contents of one liquid vitamin E capsule. Mix ingredients thoroughly and apply ointment to scars daily for at least six weeks.

Anti-ageing treatment

The astringent properties of frankincense make it a good natural ingredient in the fight against the signs of ageing. This quality helps the oil to tighten and tone the skin. Meanwhile, the abovementioned cytophylactic qualities of frankincense help to keep skin looking young and healthy by stimulating the regeneration of new skin cells. To create an anti-ageing ointment from frankincense, combine 8 drops of frankincense with 15 mL jojoba liquid wax, and the contents of one liquid vitamin E capsule. Mix thoroughly and apply ointment daily to the area of concern (e.g. crow's feet).

Immune booster

As mentioned in the previous chapter, frankincense exhibits wonderful potential when it comes to boosting the immune system. To enjoy the immune boosting benefits of frankincense, mix five drops of frankincense oil with 10mL of olive oil. Mix well to combine, and massage a small amount gently into the neck and abdomen. Repeat daily, as required.

Anti-depressant

As discussed earlier, the link between frankincense and improved mental health has been collaborated by research, suggesting that there may be substance to the ritual of burning incense in an attempt to attune one's wellbeing. One can also enjoy the mood boosting benefits of frankincense by using the essence of the synonymous incense. Perhaps the best way to administer frankincense for its anti-depressant qualities is via inhalation, through the olfactory system. This system has a close connection with the emotional center of the brain, which is also closely linked to the brain's mood and stress receptors. To utilize frankincense oil as an anti-depressant, simply add a few drops of the essence to a blank personal inhaler and administer as required.

Frankincense Oil Blend Remedies/Recipes

After having focused on the remarkable healing effect of frankincense in its own right, we will now turn to a brief collection of recipes that can be used for various therapeutic treatments. All contain frankincense as the leading active ingredient and make use of other key essential oils to deliver a wide range of therapeutic outcomes. Each blend provides clear advice on the recommended dosage and method of delivery but most may be administered in a range of other ways, if preferred. However, for those without an extensive knowledge of aromatherapy, it is recommended to stick to the ratios and delivery methods outlined below.

Please note – the ratios for the following recipes can be multiplied to make a bigger batch; however, to ensure optimal quality, blends should not be kept for longer than three months.

Acne treatment blend

Acne can be a painful and embarrassing condition which not only results in annoying and painful blemishes in the short term, but can also lead to lifelong scarring and pockmarks in more severe cases. Therefore, it is important to try and treat acne as soon as it appears, rather than letting pimples heal naturally. The following blend can be used by those with just one or two blemishes, or those suffering from a full blown breakout. It can also help to clear up oily complexions and leave skin looking toned and clear.

Thanks to its skin regeneration and scar fading properties, frankincense makes for a great base when it comes to developing an acne treatment blend. While this recipe uses frankincense as the foundation, it also includes lavender (which is an equally powerful essential oil when it comes to skin treatment) and lemon (which is great for improving skin tone). All oils also have powerful antimicrobial qualities which can help to eliminate pimple causing bacteria from the dermis. This recipe uses jojoba as a carrier which in its own right has some wonderful skin nourishing properties, with its high count of vitamins, nutrients and essential fatty acids. All of the ingredients in this blend are quite mild and should be tolerable for those with sensitive skin, however it is nonetheless recommended that a small amount of this serum is tested on a small area of the patient's skin before use.

Ingredients:

5 drops of Frankincense Oil
5 drops of Lavender Oil
3 drops of Lemon Oil
15mL Jojoba
Contents of one Vitamin E capsule

Method:

Combine ingredients in a dark glass jar and mix well to combine. Apply ointment to problem area after washing face thoroughly with a gentle cleanser. Repeat daily.

ADHD treatment blend

Millions of children and adults worldwide suffer from Attention Deficit Hyperactivity Disorder (ADHD), which is characterized by inattention and impulsivity. This can lead to poor performance at school and problems with social integration, leaving a person suffering with ADHD at a severe developmental disadvantage compared to their non-afflicted peers. However, anecdotal evidence indicates that many of the symptoms of irritability and hyperactivity that go hand in hand with ADHD can be ameliorated with a simple aromatherapy treatment. The following such remedy utilizes frankincense for its distinct ability to clear the mind and encourage focus; lavender oil, which can help to regulate levels of vital neurotransmitters important for balancing moods; and vetiver oil, which helps to instill a specific sense of groundedness in an individual.

Ingredients:
3 drops of Frankincense Oil
2 drops of Lavender Oil
2 drops of Vetiver Oil
1 Blank Inhaler

Method:
Add essential oils to blank personal inhaler. Administer inhaler as required, particularly during periods of restlessness.

Amenorrhea treatment blend

Those suffering with amenorrhea (absence of menstrual flow) can feel out of touch with their natural hormonal cycle. Monthly bleeding is a natural signal that all is well and working as it should be; conversely, the absence of a regular period can be a signal from your body that something is not quite right. This amenorrhea treatment blend can help to restore your natural cycle and can be a good complement for those who have recently ceased hormonal birth control and are looking for a return to normal hormonal function. Please note, many essential oils may act as abortifacients, and should not be used in early stages of pregnancies. The absence of menstrual flow can be an indicator of pregnancy; therefore, a pregnancy test is strongly recommended before aromatherapy treatment for amenorrhea begins. If you think you may be pregnant, or are unsure if treatment with essential oils is right for you, please seek the advice of your physician, or a licensed aromatherapist.

Ingredients:
5 drops of Frankincense Oil
4 drops of Lavender Oil
3 drops of Roman Chamomile Oil
15mL of Grapeseed Oil

Method:
Combine all ingredients in a dark glass jar and mix thoroughly. Apply a small amount of the mixture to the lower abdomen once daily. Massage gently but thoroughly.

Anti-wrinkle cream blend

Frankincense exhibits some remarkable properties when it comes to improving skin health. As mentioned above, the cytophylactic quality of frankincense helps to generate new skin cells and reduce the appearance of ageing, while the astringent nature of the essence helps to tone skin. In addition to frankincense, this blend also makes use of lemon oil, which can help to hid dark spots and blemishes, geranium oil, whose anti-inflammatory qualities can help to reduce puffiness in the face, and myrrh oil, which helps to tone and strengthen skin. The carrier use in this blend is coconut oil, which contains a large number of nutrients (including vitamin E and essential fatty acids) which are great for maintaining excellent skin health.

Ingredients:
4 drops of Frankincense Oil
3 drops of Lemon Oil
3 drops of Geranium Oil
2 drops of Myrrh Oil
15mL (about one tablespoon) of Coconut Oil

Method:
Add ingredients to a dark glass jar and mix thoroughly. Apply a moderate amount of the balm to the treatment area and massage into the skin well. For best results, apply once daily before bed.

Anti-dandruff blend

A huge number of people suffer with dry scalps and dandruff, and a large number of these use artificial anti-dandruff shampoos to treat their condition. However, not only are these treatments typically very expensive, but they can also contain potentially harmful chemicals. For example, zinc pyrithione (an active ingredient in many leading anti-dandruff shampoos) can cause skin and eye irritation in some people; on the more severe end of the spectrum, coal tar (which is banned in Canada and the European Union but can be found in some anti-dandruff products in the United States) is known to be a carcinogen and may have a toxic effect when introduced to the skin.

These concerns make an aromatherapy solution for anti-dandruff treatment a very attractive option. Not only are the ingredients in the following blend both *natural* and *safe*, the overall cost of this solution proves to be very affordable, particularly when compared to off the shelf anti-dandruff treatments. The frankincense in this remedy provides an antiseptic effect, killing of certain microbes which may be responsible for causing dandruff (while providing a lovely scent!). Meanwhile, the anti-seborrheic properties of cedarwood oil help to regulate oils in the scalp which can be a contributing factor to the skin shedding associated with dandruff. Meanwhile, the coconut oil is especially nourishing for both the scalp and the hair.

Ingredients:
5 drops of Frankincense Oil
5 drops of Cedarwood Oil
15mL (about one tablespoon) of Coconut Oil

Method:
Add ingredients to a dark glass jar and mix well to combine. Rub mixture into the hair and scalp and leave in treatment for

at least 10 minutes. For best results, apply to unwashed hair and repeat treatment every other day.

Arthritis treatment blend

The crippling pain of arthritis demands effective treatment of both the symptoms and the source of discomfort. Fortunately, the following remedy offers both. The frankincense oil therein offer strong anti-inflammatory power, as well as pain relief, while German chamomile and helichrysum have also been shown to provide a potent anti-inflammatory effect. Olive oil, as the carrier oil in this blend, has in its own right shown to be effective in treating the pain and inflammation associated with arthritis.

Ingredients:
4 drops of Frankincense Oil
3 drops of German Chamomile Oil
3 drops of Helichrysum Oil
15mL of Olive Oil

Method:
Combine ingredients in a dark glass jar and shake well. Apply a moderate amount of ointment to the affected area, massaging thoroughly. Administer treatment daily for best results.

Asthma treatment blend

Asthma is a very common inflammatory disease which affects the normal function of the body's respiratory system. During an 'asthma attack', the sufferer's airways become inflamed and swollen, narrowing the area through which air passes to the lungs. This can be an incredibly unpleasant experience at best, and life-threatening at worst. The following asthma treatment blend makes use of the anti-inflammatory properties of frankincense, which is complemented by the soothing, anti-inflammatory and antispasmodic properties of lavender and peppermint.

Ingredients:
4 drops of Frankincense Oil
4 drops of Lavender Oil
3 drops of Peppermint Oil
Room diffuser

Method:
Add oils to a room diffuser. Administer treatment as required. Avoid direct inhalation as this may trigger irritation and lead to an asthma attack.

Bad breath remedy blend

For centuries, people have chewed away at frankincense resin to help eliminate bad breath and as a way of maintaining satisfactory oral health. This effect is possible thanks to the strong antiseptic and antimicrobial qualities of frankincense oil (supported by its pleasant flavor and aroma). The following remedy can be used to help fight persistent bad breath using the method of gargling. Aside from the main ingredient of frankincense, this blend also contains peppermint which, aside from having a particularly refreshing taste and scent, also exhibits a potent antibacterial effect, killing the germs that can cause bad breath.

Ingredients:
5 drops of Frankincense Oil
4 drops of Peppermint Oil
1 glass of Water

Method:
Add oils to glass of water and stir to combine. Take one mouthful at a time and gargle with solution for 10-15 seconds. Spit out the solution in a sink. Repeat process with remaining solution until finished. For best results, apply treatment twice daily after brushing teeth.

Bell's Palsy treatment blend

Bell's palsy is a condition whereby the muscles or nerves on one side of the face become temporarily and partially paralyzed. Although the exact cause of Bell's palsy is unclear, it is thought to be the result of an inflammation of the main group of nerves responsible for controlling facial movement. The onset of the condition is normally very sudden, often occurring overnight and without warning. And while the effects of Bell's palsy are generally temporary (normally lasting for just a few weeks), it can be an uncomfortable and disquieting condition for the sufferer. The following remedy can help to speed recovery from the symptoms of Bell's palsy, restoring healthy nerve function sooner than without treatment.

Please note that although there is no direct link between stroke and Bell's palsy, the two share similar symptoms; as such, self-diagnosis of Bell's palsy should not be made. If an occurrence of Bell's palsy is suspected, assessment by a physician should be sought immediately.

Ingredients:
4 drops of Frankincense Oil
4 drops of Helichrysum Oil
2 drops of Peppermint Oil
15mL of Grapeseed Oil

Method:
Combine ingredients in a dark glass jar and mix thoroughly. Apply ointment to the affected area once daily before bed.

Broken bone repairing blend

Remarkably, frankincense can prove to be an effective treatment for encouraging the healing of bone fractures. Although it may not directly speed the fusion of the break itself, it can help to reduce inflammation in the area surrounding the fracture, which can create a more optimal environment for the bone to mend. Additionally, frankincense can help to relieve the pain associated with a broken bone. Of course, all suspected bone fractures should be checked out by a trained physician in the first instance. This blend should be used as a supplementary treatment to aid the healing of small, minor fractures (such as a broken toe, for example).

Ingredients:
10 drops of Frankincense Oil
5 drops of Wintergreen Oil
5 drops of Helichrysum Oil

Method:
Add oils to a warm bath. Submerge affected area in bath water for at least 20 minutes. Repeat daily until fracture has healed.

Bronchitis treatment blend

As many of the symptoms of bronchitis relate to inflammation of the bronchial tubes, frankincense can make a good treatment for those suffering with bronchial infection. As discussed earlier, frankincense has a potent anti-inflammatory effect which can help to reduce swelling in the airways. Meanwhile, the antibacterial effect of the oil can help to fight microbial infection of the lungs. Finally, as an expectorant, frankincense also works to clear the lungs of mucus. This blend also benefits from the antibacterial effect of eucalyptus oil and the soothing effect of lemon.

Ingredients:
6 drops of Frankincense Oil
4 drops of Eucalyptus Oil
4 drops of Lemon Oil
15mL of Grapeseed Oil

Method:
Combine ingredients in a dark glass jar and mix thoroughly. Apply ointment to the chest and massage gently into the area. Reapply every 4-6 hours.

Cancer treatment blend

As discussed in earlier chapters, there has been quite a lot of research conducted in recent times as to the efficacy of frankincense as a treatment for the healing of some cancers. Although a robust anti-cancer treatment is yet to be developed with frankincense as the active ingredient, links have certainly been identified – both anecdotally and scientifically – between the administration of frankincense oil and the reduction of some cancers. Furthermore, it is unknown exactly which cancers frankincense may target, although research has indicated a positive effect when it comes to reducing a number of different cancers, including pancreatic, bladder and ovarian carcinoma cells. For these reasons, aromatherapy treatment with frankincense should not be relied upon as a cure-all for cancer patients but instead should be looked to as a complementary therapy to be used *in addition to* traditional cancer treatments. This is reflected by the fact that this blend contains ingredients that are aimed at providing cancer treatment *support,* targeting the symptoms associated with some cancers. Advice should be sought from a licensed physician before beginning any course of aromatherapy treatment aimed at addressing cancer, particularly as some essential oils may inhibit the effectivity of other cancer treatments (such as chemotherapy).

Ingredients:
8 drops of Frankincense Oil
4 drops of Helichrysum Oil
3 drops of Peppermint Oil
3 drops of Basil Oil
15mL of Grapeseed Oil

Method:
Combine ingredients in a dark glass jar and mix well. Apply ointment to the neck and abdomen twice daily. If possible, combine with lymphatic drainage massage treatment.

Circulation boosting blend

For those suffering from poor circulation, this remedy (which contains frankincense as its main active ingredient) can help to restore normal blood flow throughout the body. Discoloration of the fingers or toes, tingling or numbness in the extremities, and dizziness or light-headedness, can all be indications of poor circulation. This treatment can help to restore normal circulation within a matter of days, with regular application.

Ingredients:
5 drops of Frankincense
4 drops of Geranium Oil
2 drops of Ginger Oil
15mL of Sweet Almond Oil

Method:
Combine ingredients in a dark glass jar and mix well. Apply ointment to affected area, daily before bed.

Congestion treatment blend

A stuffy or blocked nose is a relatively common occurrence and can be a rather unpleasant experience, often leading to disrupted breathing and sleeping patterns. Fortunately, the congestion from a cold, flu or sinus infection can be effectively treated with a blend containing frankincense. The anti-inflammatory properties of the oil help to mitigate swelling of the sinus passages, while the antimicrobial effect of the essence can help to kill any infection that may be causing the congestion. Additionally, the expectorant property of frankincense helps to draw out mucus.

Ingredients:
4 drops of Frankincense Oil
4 drops of Eucalyptus Oil
2 drops of Peppermint Oil
Steam basin

Method:
Add ingredients, including boiling water, to a steam basin. Place head over basin and cover with a towel, taking care to avoid skin contact with steam. Take long, deep breaths, inhaling through the nose. Repeat treatment as needed.

Deodorant blend

With its pleasant, fragrant aroma and antimicrobial properties, frankincense can make an excellent foundation for a great natural deodorant. Most of us thoughtlessly apply deodorant to our bodies every day, most of which contain chemicals and metals which can have an unknown effect on our overall wellbeing. Using a deodorant made entirely from natural ingredients can give us peace of mind that we aren't applying a potential harmful substance to our armpits on a daily basis!

Ingredients:
10 drops of Frankincense Oil
10 drops of Lavender Oil
4 drops of Myrrh Oil
¼ cup of Baking Soda

Method:
Combine ingredients in a wide-mouthed jar and stir well with a spoon or spatula until a thoroughly mixed. Take a small amount of the mixture and pat onto dry armpits. For best results, use after showering.

Detoxification blend

With its ability to act as a natural diuretic, frankincense can help to flush the body of impurities through stimulating the function of the renal system. With the kidneys operating at full function, toxins are expunged from the body through urine and one can begin to enjoy the benefits of detoxification. This blend also makes use of lemon oil, which has proven to exhibit excellent detoxification powers in its own right, as well as lavender, which stimulates both hepatic and renal detoxification.

Ingredients:
5 drops of Frankincense Oil
5 drops of Lemon Oil
5 drops of Lavender Oil
15mL of Grapeseed Oil

Method:
Combine ingredients in a dark glass jar and stir thoroughly. Apply mixture to abdomen, massaging the area well.

Exhaustion relief blend

As discussed above, perhaps one of the leading properties of frankincense oil is the effect that it has on the mind. In this blend, frankincense's remarkable ability to focus the mind can help to bring us 'back to earth' when experience intense exhaustion. The peppermint and basil in this blend further augment the power of frankincense, and make for a stimulating, focusing pick-me-up.

Ingredients:
3 drops of Frankincense Oil
2 drops of Peppermint Oil
2 drops of Basil Oil
Blank inhaler

Method:
Add oils to the cotton swab of a blank personal inhaler. Use when bouts of tiredness or exhaustion arise; administer as often as required.

Hair treatment blend

As with its ability to restore skin to optimum health, so too can frankincense instill hair with a healthy luster and shine. The following treatment works particularly well for dry or damaged hair, but can be used for good results with all hair types.

Ingredients:
6 drops of Frankincense Oil
4 drops of Myrrh Oil
5 drops of Lavender Oil
15mL of Jojoba

Method:
Combine ingredients in a dark glass jar and shake well to combine. Apply treatment to hair and leave in for 10 minutes. Rinse treatment from hair with warm water. For best results, apply treatment twice weekly.

Hemorrhoid treatment blend

There is perhaps nothing more irritating or uncomfortable than the pain and itchiness associated with hemorrhoids. To explain how the following remedy works, we must first understand exactly what a hemorrhoid is. Hemorrhoids (or 'piles') are in fact swollen blood vessels that occur either internally or externally (in relation to the anus), and typically arise due to excessive straining during a bowel movement, or during pregnancy. They can cause bleeding, itchiness and pain and discomfort during a bowel movement. In some more severe cases, they can even lead to infection. Although piles normally remedy themselves after some time, in some cases they can persist for weeks, months or years.

The following blend offers relief from the discomfort of hemorrhoids and speeds the healing process. Here, frankincense oil has the effect of acting as an anti-inflammatory, helping the blood vessels return to their natural state. Lavender has a similar effect, while adding a strong soothing element to the mixture, while geranium also acts as a powerful anti-inflammatory. The use of coconut oil as the carrier serves two purposes: first, it helps to improve the health of the skin in the area with its rich array of nutrients and second, it makes for easy application to the affected area.

Ingredients:
4 drops of Frankincense Oil
4 drops of Lavender Oil
3 drops of Geranium Oil
15mL (about one tablespoon) of Coconut Oil

Method:
Combine ingredients in a dark glass jar and mix well. Wash the affected area with warm water and pat dry. Apply ointment to the affected area. For best results, apply daily until hemorrhoids have cleared.

Inflammation treatment blend

As a potent anti-inflammatory, frankincense can be used in its own right in the treatment of conditions where inflammation occurs. However, the following blend – making use of the complementary anti-inflammatory properties of lavender and thyme – is a real powerhouse when it comes to reducing pain and swelling for all manner of inflammation related conditions.

Ingredients:
5 drops of Frankincense Oil
5 drops of Lavender Oil
5 drops of Thyme Oil
10mL of Olive Oil

Method:
Combine ingredients in a dark glass jar and shake well to combine. Apply a moderate amount of the tincture topically to the affected area, massaging gently into the skin. Apply as required.

Insect bite treatment blend

A must during the warm months in which biting insects tend to swarm, the following blend is an effective treatment when it comes to alleviating the pain or itch of a bug bite. With its pain relief, antimicrobial and anti-inflammatory properties, frankincense can provide relief from insect bites while helping to kill any germs introduced to the skin by the bug and its bite. This blend also makes use of peppermint, which help to cool the sting/itch of a bite, as well as lavender, which soothes the skin. Soothing aloe vera rounds out this remedy as a complete insect bite relief treatment.

Ingredients:
5 drops of Frankincense Oil
5 drops of Lavender Oil
2 drops of Peppermint Oil
15mL of Aloe Vera Gel

Method:
Combine ingredients in a dark glass jar and mix well. Dab a small amount of the ointment on insect bites for quick relief from pain and irritation.

Insomnia treatment blend

Insomnia is a condition that affects millions of people worldwide, and can be extremely disruptive when it comes to living a normal life. Not only can a lack of sleep lead to us feeling general tiredness and malaise throughout the course of our day, but it can also result in significant health problems, such as high blood pressure and stroke. Thankfully, relief can come with a course of aromatherapy treatment, including with the remedy outlined below. This blend makes use of frankincense as its main active ingredient, thanks to its ability to calm the mind, and is complemented by lavender and roman chamomile.

Ingredients:
4 drops of Frankincense Oil
4 drops of Lavender Oil
4 drops of Roman Chamomile Oil
Room diffuser

Method:
Add oils to room diffuser, and focus on breathing deeply for 10 minutes. For best results, carry out treatment about 30-40 minutes before bedtime.

Irritable bowel syndrome treatment blend

Irritable bowel syndrome can vary in its severity, from relatively mild discomfort to severe cramping and diarrhea. The following blend can help to provide relief from the symptoms of irritable bowel syndrome, which can be highly disruptive in living a normal, day to day life. As a carminative, digestive and anti-inflammatory, the frankincense in this blend works by reducing gas and bloating associated with IBS, encouraging healthy digestive function, and reducing swelling and inflammation in the digestive system.

Ingredients:
5 drops of Frankincense Oil
5 drops of Lavender Oil
1 drop of Ginger Oil
1 drop of Peppermint Oil
15mL of Grapeseed Oil

Method:
Combine ingredients in a dark glass and mix thoroughly. Apply a moderate amount of the treatment blend to the abdomen, massaging the area gently. Administer as required.

Jet lag blend

Thanks once again to frankincense's ability to focus and calm the mind, it makes the great centerpiece of a remedy for jet lag. With international travel more common than ever, many of us have experienced jet lag – that feeling of our body being in one place and our mind remaining on the other side of the world. Thankfully, this remedy can go a long way towards helping us to feel human again after a long haul flight. And thanks to the fact that it can be prepared ahead of time and tucked away into our carry-on luggage, we can be prepared to fight jet lag anytime, anywhere!

Ingredients:
3 drops of Frankincense Oil
2 drops of Peppermint Oil
2 drops of Bergamot Oil
1 Blank inhaler

Method:
Apply oils to cotton pad of blank inhaler. Administer every few hours during long haul travel, or as required.

Memory improvement blend

All of us have suffered some sort of memory loss at one time or another, whether it's forgetting a name or where we put the car keys. As we age, our memory generally deteriorates even further. Indeed, memory loss can rapidly move from benign, occasional forgetfulness, to chronic failure to recall the most fundamental details about our own lives that is a characteristic of dementia or Alzheimer's disease. Although we may be a long way from discovering a cure for the latter, more severe example of memory loss, we can use the power of aromatherapy to encourage memory recall.

Another of frankincense's remarkable and distinct properties can be seen in its connection with memory enhancement. Its ability to focus the mind when introduced via the olfactory system is second to none in the world of aromatherapy. What's more, scent has been proved to be the sense most closely affiliated with memory, and for this reason this treatment is best administered via inhalation. The frankincense in this blend is complemented by rosemary, which has equally strong links to improving mental recall, along with invigorating peppermint oil.

Ingredients:
5 drops of Frankincense Oil
5 drops of Rosemary Oil
3 drops of Peppermint Oil
Room diffuser/Blank inhaler

Method:
Add oils to room diffuser or blank inhaler. Administer periodically (every two to three days) to improve general memory function and recall.

Mouth ulcer treatment blend

Mouth ulcers – also known as *canker sores* – are both painful and annoying. These sores can appear in and around the mouth, typically on the inner cheek, lip or gums. They can pop up at any time, often due to burning or biting of the sensitive membranes inside the mouth, or sometimes simply due to a weak immune system. Frankincense can be a great agent for treating mouth ulcers for a few reasons. First, its anti-inflammatory and analgesic properties help to reduce swelling and pain, making a sore more bearable. Second, the antiseptic qualities of frankincense help to keep the ulcer and the area surrounding it free from infection. Third, the cytophylactic properties of frankincense help to repair skin cells inside the mouth and encourage the growth of healthy tissue. The following blend also makes use of peppermint, which freshens the breath and helps to kill germs, and myrrh, which also targets pain and inflammation.

Ingredients:
4 drops of Frankincense Oil
2 drops of Myrrh Oil
2 drops of Peppermint Oil
Glass of Water

Method:
Add oils to glass of water and stir well. Taking one mouthful of solution at a time, rinse inside of the mouth thoroughly (for about 15 seconds) before spitting into sink. Continue with the remaining solution until finished. Perform treatment once daily after brushing teeth until ulcer(s) have dissipated.

Parkinson's disease treatment blend

Parkinson's disease is a degenerative brain condition the affects the ability to control voluntary movement. It can affect the sufferer in a number of different ways, from impairing basic motor functions needed for day to day function, to making articulated speech practically impossible. In its later stages, the disease can induce behavioral and psychological problems including depression, emotional dissonance and dementia. There is no cure for Parkinson's disease, although millions of research dollars have been spent in its pursuit. Around one million Americans are thought to suffer from Parkinson's disease.

Although aromatherapy cannot cure Parkinson's disease, it can provide much needed relief from its symptoms. In the following blend, frankincense both helps to reduce inflammation in the brain and foster mental clarity. Geranium complements the anti-inflammatory effect of frankincense, while vetiver oil may help to reduce tremors.

Ingredients:
5 drops of Frankincense Oil
4 drops of Geranium Oil
3 drops of Vetiver Oil
Room diffuser

Method:
Add oils to room diffuser and breathe deeply for at least 30 minutes. Administer treatment once daily on an ongoing basis for best results.

Seizure treatment blend

The experience of a seizure can be a terribly frightening one, both for the sufferer and for those around them. Perhaps the most terrifying thing about seizures is that they can come completely out of the blue, making them practically impossible to pre-empt. Meanwhile, the cause of seizures can be many and varied. Often, the cause is irregular nerve function due to epilepsy; however, seizures can also be a symptom of a more serious, underlying pathology, such as a brain tumor. For this reason, the occurrence of a seizure should be immediately followed up by a thorough examination by a physician. In some severe cases, a doctor may prescribe anti-seizure medication (which should not be substituted by the following treatment).

Those who have a family history of seizures, or have experienced seizures in the past, may administer the following remedy periodically to try and minimize the chance of a seizure occurring. The frankincense in this blend, as discussed above, has a generally positive effect on brain health and may work in this instance by reducing brain inflammation. Meanwhile, lemon and orange oils have also been shown to have a positive anti-seizure effect. As outlined above, please seek the advice of a physician before beginning this treatment.

Ingredients:
5 drops of Frankincense Oil
3 drops of Lemon Oil
3 drops of Orange Oil
15mL (about one tablespoon) of Coconut Oil

Method:
Add ingredients to a dark glass jar and mix until combined. Apply a small amount of ointment to temples twice daily.

Scar/stretch mark fading blend

Unsightly scars and stretch marks can be both embarrassing and damaging to one's confidence. Fortunately, those of us suffering with scars, stretch marks or any kind of unsightly skin blemishes can apply the following treatment for good cosmetic effect. Once again, frankincense's cytophylactic skin regeneration properties come to the rescue here as the backbone of a treatment for improving the appearance of scars or stretch marks. Lavender, too, is particularly friendly to the skin, with excellent healing properties (discussed in detail in the preceding book in this series), while neroli can also yield positive results in scar improvement. Meanwhile, the rosehip seed oil and liquid vitamin E provide additional nourishment for damaged skin.

Ingredients:
5 drops of Frankincense Oil
4 drops of Lavender Oil
3 drops of Neroli Oil
15mL Rosehip Seed Oil
Contents of one Vitamin E capsule

Method:
Add ingredients to dark glass jar and mix well. Apply ointment liberally to affected area and massage well. For best results, apply daily. Some improvement should be observed after a few weeks.

Urinary tract infection blend

Recurring urinary tract infections (UTIs) can be an absolute nightmare. They can seemingly spring up out of nowhere, leaving you doubled over in pain and constantly running to the toilet. What's more, serious UTIs, if left unchecked, can lead to complications from secondary infections. The following treatment helps to clear and prevent UTIs, and will make chronic infections a thing of the past. In this blend, frankincense's antibacterial, analgesic and anti-inflammatory qualities help to attack the infection, and reduce pain and swelling. Additionally, the diuretic function of the essence helps to flush the kidneys and the urinary tract of infection. These properties are complemented by the inclusion of oregano and lemon.

Ingredients:
5 drops of Frankincense Oil
4 drops of Lemon Oil
3 drops of Oregano Oil
10mL of Grapeseed Oil

Method:
Combine ingredients in a dark glass jar and shake well to mix. Add a moderate amount of the ointment to the abdomen and massage the area thoroughly. For best results, apply daily for a week.

Wart treatment blend

Warts come in many different shapes and sizes, but all have one thing in common – they are notoriously difficult to eradicate. These small, approximately circular skin growths are typically caused by a virus (known as the human papilloma virus – or *HPV*) which affects the top layer (or 'dermis') of the skin. Although warts typically appear on the hands and feet, they can occur almost anywhere on the body. The following blend – containing frankincense, oregano and lavender – is particular effective when it comes to treating and eliminating practically all types of wart. As warts normally originate from a HPV infection, it is important to attempt to treat this underlying cause. This blend, therefore, has strong anti-viral properties and can target HPV successfully, while the other properties of each of these oils help the skin to remain healthy and regenerate new, normal tissue.

Ingredients:
4 drops of Frankincense Oil
2 drops of Oregano Oil
2 drops of Lavender Oil
10mL of Sweet Almond Oil

Method:
Combine ingredient in a dark glass jar and shake well. Apply a small amount of the mixture to the affected area and leave to soak into skin. Administer treatment three times daily until wart has cleared.

Wound cleanser blend

Cuts, grazes, scrapes, lacerations – all of these and many more different types of wounds will occur in the home over a few years, *especially* when there are children in the family! Therefore, having a natural and effective way to clean and treat wounds in the home is of paramount importance. The following blend combines essential oils with powerful antiseptic and antimicrobial properties, along with the soothing aloe vera gel, to make an unbeatable, all-purpose wound cleanser. Please note – severe wounds may require urgent medical attention.

Ingredients:
5 drops of Frankincense Oil
5 drops of Lavender Oil
3 drops of Eucalyptus Oil
10mL Aloe Vera Gel

Method:
Combine ingredients in a dark glass jar and mix thoroughly. After rinsing wound under cool, clean water, apply a moderate amount of the wound cleanser to the affected area. Leave wound open to breathe and repeat treatment twice a day until injury has healed.

Conclusion

There is perhaps no other essential oil that has been imbued with such value as frankincense: from ancient times, lasting through to today. Frankincense, quite literally, has been a prized commodity for millennia. This is of course thanks, in part, to the highly specific climactic conditions required to grow the species of tree from which precious frankincense resin is harvested. As with all of the world's commodities, the rarity of frankincense has a direct correlation with value. In another way, frankincense has proved its worth with regards to the impressive healing properties that it has proved to exhibit. It has been believed – and has been shown – to have an immense power over the mind and body, fascinating healers of different eras with its restorative effect. Even today, frankincense's secrets have not been fully exposed; its association with the remission of cancer, for example, has just begun to be explored by the scientific world. Indeed, the value of frankincense is perhaps grounded partly in the enigmatic and seemingly magical qualities of the essence, with the depths of its capacity to heal remaining partially shrouded in mystery.

This book has attempted to somewhat remove this shroud and makes an effort to summarize the collective knowledge on frankincense in one convenient location. From the chemical constituency of the essence of frankincense, to the therapeutic properties attributed to frankincense oil, this guide has made efforts to highlight the therapeutic power of frankincense and make it accessible to those who wish to not only learn more about this remarkable commodity, but also put this knowledge to practical use. From theory to application, both novice and master aromatherapist can take something from this guide to complement their pursuit of alternative healing methods using essential oils and, more specifically, the wonderful and enigmatic frankincense oil.

Check Out My Other Essential Oils Books!

Simply click on the books title or type the links below into your web browser. Alternatively you can search for "Amy Joyson" in the Kindle Store.

Essential Oils: The Complete Guide:
http://www.amazon.com/gp/product/B00T12QLW4

Essential Oils Massage Techniques:
http://www.amazon.com/gp/product/B00VITFIQI

Essential Oils For Allergies:
http://www.amazon.com/gp/product/B00X6ANQKM

Essential Oils For Dogs:
http://www.amazon.com/gp/product/B00XSDE6N8

Lavender Essential Oil:
http://www.amazon.com/gp/product/B00WTBTHPC

2 FREE eBooks for you!

Guys, thanks so much for reading my book. I truly hope it served as a great introduction to frankincense essential oil. As a token of appreciation I have prepared two free ebooks for you. Here is a bit of information about them!

The 10 Most Important Essential Oils

In this book we delve deep into the uses and applications of the ten essential oils that I consider to be the most 'essential'. For each oil I explain the key health benefits, teach you the therapeutic applications and provide specific safety precaution. I include one of my most useful remedies for each of the oils as well. So you will receive a deep knowledge of ten essential oils and ten brilliant remedies for free! It is a 10k word eBook, the same length as this one!

When you receive this ebook you will also receive a couple of emails from me a week containing even more information about the essential oils! I will endeavour to give you at least 5 recipes or remedies per week and also provide you with some great information on the lesser known essential oils.

Type this link into a web browser: http://bit.ly/1EuHgyn

The Ultimate Guide To Vitamins

This is another wonderful 10k word ebook that has been made available to you through my publisher, Valerian Press. As a health conscious person you should be well aware of the uses and health benefits of each of the vitamins that should make up our diet. This book gives you an easy to understand, scientific explanation of the vitamin followed by the recommended daily dosage. It then highlights all the important health benefits of each vitamin. A list of the best sources of each vitamin is provided and you are also given some actionable next steps for each vitamin to make sure you are utilizing the information!

As well as receiving the free ebooks you will also be sent a weekly stream of free ebooks, again from my publishing company Valerian Press. You can expect to receive at least a new, free ebook each and every week. Sometimes you might receive a massive 10 free books in a week!

Type this link into a web browser: http://bit.ly/1EuHgyn

About The Author

Hey there! I'm Amy Joyson, a lifelong student of holistic and alternative medicine. My journey began as far back as I can remember, my mother, a practicing aromatherapist, taught me value of natural remedies as a youngster. I don't think I could imagine a life without the essential oils if I tried, they are just so important to me. I am passionate about sharing their value with as many people as possible, which led me to writing my books. If you have read any of my books I truly hope they have added value to your life and I thank you with all my heart for trusting in me.

Outside of being an author, I work as a personal trainer. Employing my deep knowledge of alternative treatments has enabled me to provide outstanding results for all of my clients!

In my spare time you will often find me lounging in my hammock reading the latest aromatherapy magazine or romantic fiction novel. I have a soft spot for true romance! I aim to meditate at least once a day, and practice yoga 5 times a week. My biggest hobby however is exploring the beautiful world that we live in. Next on my hit list is Iceland, there is something seriously alluring about that island.

Valerian Press

At Valerian Press we have three key beliefs.

Providing outstanding value: We believe in enriching all of our customers' lives, doing everything we can to ensure the best experience.

Championing new talent: We believe in showcasing the worlds emerging talent by giving them the platform to grow.

Simplicity and efficiency: We understand how valuable your time is. Our products are stream-lined and consist only of what you want. You will find no fluff with us.

We hope you have enjoyed reading Amy's guide to Frankincense Essential Oil

We would love to offer you a regular supply of our free and discounted books. We cover a huge range of non-fiction genres; diet and cookbooks, health and fitness, alternative and holistic medicine, spirituality and plenty more.

All you need to do is simply type this link into your web browser: http://bit.ly/18hmup4

Free Preview of "Lavender Essential Oil"

Lavender oil is derived from the steam distillation of the plant of the same name (typically, the *Lavandula angustifolia* species of the lavender genus), which is believed to be native to the Mediterranean region of Southern Europe and North Africa. Lavender is classified as a flowering herb and is a member of the mint family. It has enjoyed its position as a revered medicinal herb for some thousands of years, with evidence of popular use in nearly all major ancient Eurasian cultures. The Ancient Egyptians are known to have used lavender in the preparation of tinctures for use during the embalming process, while it was also found to be a key ingredient in the herb, spice and sawdust blend used to stuff mummies and aid with their preservation. Additionally, lavender was commonly used in Egypt in various cosmetic preparations. The Greeks also used lavender prolifically, however, their usage of the flower took on a more therapeutic bent than the Egyptians. There, the plant was used as a cure-all remedy for various psychosomatic conditions, from insomnia to insanity and beyond. The contemporary name for the plant is possibly derived from the Latin *lavare*, or 'to wash', which hints at the typical Roman usage of the flower. (Another potential etymological source comes from the Latin word *livindulo*, meaning 'livid or bluish'). Typically, lavender was used as an aromatic by the Romans to scent their baths, dwellings and clothing. Lavender was also used cosmetically by wealthy patricians throughout the Empire as a perfume and treatment for the skin and hair.

Whatever the true origin of the present day name of the plant, lavender has maintained a long association with cleanliness and purification, from ancient times through to the modern era. There is an abundance of evidence of a strong connection between domestic cleanliness and the usage of lavender as a purificant across cultures; here again, the etymological connection is clear. The word 'launder' is believed to have evolved from *lavendre,* which is the Old French word for the same term. Indeed, the use of lavender in instilling freshness in clothing and linens via special lavender infused washes was a common practice used by 'launderers' throughout history, with evidence of this practice existing across a number of different cultures. The appeal of lavender for use as a cleaning agent is certainly understandable; not only does the strong, yet pleasant scent of the flower mask any potentially offensive odors, but fabrics (and flesh) treated with lavender would have been noted to have kept cleaner for a longer period than those effects and persons treated without it. This would have seemed like a rather magical property in pre-modern times; however, we now know this attribute is due to the antimicrobial effect of lavender, which would work to kill bugs that generated nasty smells.

Yet, it is not merely the power of lavender to clean that has given this special plant such a revered place in history. The medicinal and healing properties of lavender have also long been observed and held in high esteem. We have already seen how the Ancient Greeks used lavender to treat various health related conditions. Interestingly, however, this tendency to use lavender for medicinal purposes is one that endured for centuries and was again a practice that permeated throughout various cultures. For example, grave robbers during the 17th century proliferation of the Bubonic Plague throughout France are rumoured to have maintained their good health (despite the extremely dangerous nature of their work) by washing in a powerful disinfectant known as 'Four Thieves Vinegar'. As one might expect, one of the principal ingredients in this prophylactic against one of history's deadliest diseases, was humble lavender. Though the narrative of this story likely has its foundations in folkloric mythology, there is colloquial evidence of lavender being used around this time to ward off the insidious 'Black Death'.

Lavender also has strong links to the modern foundation of the practice of aromatherapy. In fact, it is often viewed as the 'first oil' of the discipline, both in chronological and taxonomical terms. In the case of the former, it can be linked to a very particular moment in the history of aromatherapy, when Rene Gatefossé (a renowned French chemist) stumbled upon the remarkable healing properties of lavender oil. As with many great scientific discoveries throughout history, Gatefossé's encounter with lavender oil as an agent for healing was largely serendipitous. During an unrelated scientific experiment gone awry, the chemist received severe burns to his hands and arms. In a moment of desperation, he plunged his hands into the nearest available solution that could likely provide relief to his injuries – a large vat of lavender oil. Although Gatefossé is understood to have not been fully aware of the healing potential of lavender oil at the time, the remarkable qualities of the essence soon became apparent to him, as his injuries began to heal at an unexpectedly rapid rate. This experience soon saw Gatefossé begin a further scientific exploration of the therapeutic qualities of other essential oils. This eventually led the French chemist to become known as the 'father of aromatherapy', and one of the leading figures in driving a renewed interest in the remedial potential of essential oils in modern times.

However, it isn't simply because of its place in history that lavender is viewed with such pre-eminence in the world of aromatherapy. In taxonomical terms, there are many arguments for placing lavender oil at the top of the tree, especially when it comes to the oil's long list of remarkable therapeutic properties. As we have seen from the above historical accounts, lavender exhibits some very powerful antimicrobial qualities. Its prolific usage in cleaning and personal hygiene across various cultures is not coincidental;

rather, the antibacterial effect of lavender that can help to kill bugs and germs is also effective in eliminating nasty odors. Additionally, its attribution as a key ingredient in the plague-fighting 'Four Thieves Vinegar' provides another hint at the oil's strong antimicrobial properties. While most modern users of lavender are unlikely to need to recruit lavender for use as a prophylactic against the Black Death, it nonetheless has a number of therapeutic applications for the remedy of a number of bacteria related complaints. Although its use as a prophylactic against disease in pre-modern times would perhaps have had more of a basis in mysticism than science, we know today that lavender can be relied upon as a powerful natural antiseptic. We will discuss all of these therapeutic attributes of lavender in more detail in later chapters.

As we can see from this brief introduction to lavender, perhaps no other oil has been more influential or remarkable in its consistent and common use among different cultures throughout history. Its range of uses has varied over time from disinfectant and deodorant, to antiseptic and relaxant, and many more. Today, lavender remains immensely popular, both for its unique fragrance and for its plethora of therapeutic qualities when used in aromatherapy treatments. With a broad understanding of the historical significance of lavender oil, we will take a detailed look in the following chapter at the properties that are responsible for bestowing such a mighty reputation upon this humble plant.

To grab this complete guide to lavender essential oil simply type this link into your web browser:

http://www.amazon.com/gp/product/B00WTBTHPC

Or search for Amy Joyson on Amazon!

CPSIA information can be obtained
at www.ICGtesting.com
Printed in the USA
BVHW01s0810040218
507175BV00020B/295/P